LYN MARSHALL'S

YOGACISE

The 'no-sweat' exercise programme for the 90s

BBC Books

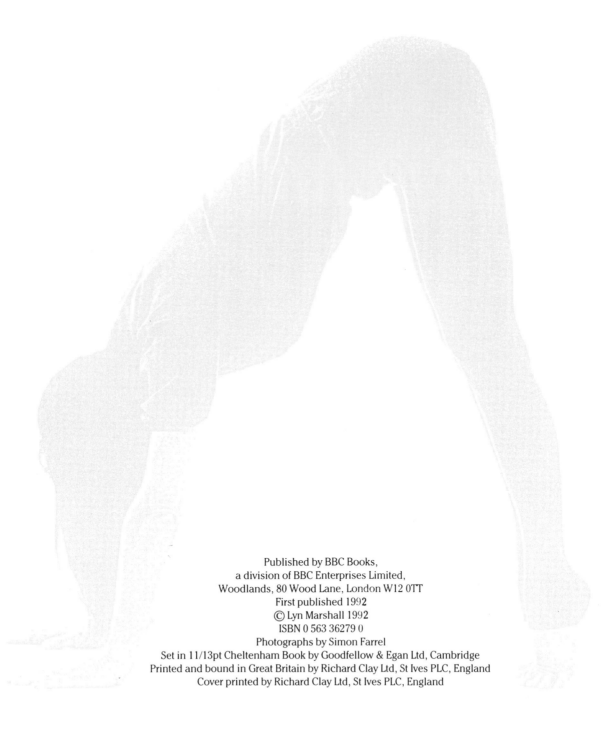

Published by BBC Books,
a division of BBC Enterprises Limited,
Woodlands, 80 Wood Lane, London W12 0TT
First published 1992
© Lyn Marshall 1992
ISBN 0 563 36279 0
Photographs by Simon Farrel
Set in 11/13pt Cheltenham Book by Goodfellow & Egan Ltd, Cambridge
Printed and bound in Great Britain by Richard Clay Ltd, St Ives PLC, England
Cover printed by Richard Clay Ltd, St Ives PLC, England

CONTENTS

~~~~~~~~~~~~~~~

Introduction   7

How Yogacise was born   8
What is Yogacise?   9
Can anybody do Yogacise?   10
Is Yogacise safe?   10
Is there an age limit for Yogacise?   12
What are the physical benefits of Yogacise?   13
What are the mental and emotional benefits of
    Yogacise?   14
When should I do Yogacise and for how long?   15
Where should I do Yogacise?   15
What should I wear to practise?   16
Why music?   16
On your own or in a group?   17
Yogacise for life   17
How to use this book   18
Practice introduction   19

Standing Movements

Yogacise Standing Breath   21
Yogacise Standing Reach-Up (single arm)   22
Yogacise Standing Reach-Up (both arms)   24
Yogacise Side Slide   26
Yogacise Triangle   28
Yogacise Forward Bend   30
Yogacise Squat   32

Kneeling Movements

Yogacise Kneeling Reach-Up   34
Yogacise Sit Down   36
Yogacise Kneeling Back Wave   37
Yogacise Uncoil   38

Yogacise Cat   40
Yogacise 'V'   42

Sitting Movements
Yogacise Seated Reach-Up   44
Yogacise Head to Knees   46
Yogacise Shoulder Twist   48
Yogacise Seated Back Wave   50
Yogacise Shoulder Rotations   51
Yogacise Arm Circling   52
Yogacise Elbow Bends   53
Yogacise Head Roll   54
Yogacise Eye Rotations   56
Yogacise Finger Spread   58
Yogacise Fists   59
Yogacise Finger Pulls   60
Yogacise Foot Work   61

Lying Movements
Yogacise Lying Breath   62
Yogacise Stretch   64
Yogacise Cobra   66
Yogacise Coil   68
Yogacise Fish   70
Yogacise Hip Push   72
Yogacise Leg Work (single leg)   74
Yogacise Leg Work (both legs)   76
Yogacise Side Raise   78
Yogacise Hip Twist   80
Yogacise Locust   82
Yogacise Sit Up – Lie Down   84

Yogacise Routines   86
Yogacise and Pregnancy   90
Glossary   91

ABOUT THE AUTHOR

~~~~~~~~~~~~~~~~~~

Lyn Marshall has been successfully teaching her unique form of exercise, relaxation and stress management for over twenty years. She has starred in five television series on yoga and has written a number of best-selling books. She also lectures and teaches privately.

Lyn's style of exercise is a series of carefully worked out slow, gentle stretches. These movements are not only effective in slimming, firming and toning the body from head to toe but, at the same time, they are also extremely pleasant and relaxing to do.

Yogacise is Lyn's latest fitness programme and it combines a new, ultra gentle form of yoga with music. 'It is', she says, 'the no-effort exercise,' and is specially designed for people who want easily and enjoyably to improve their bodies and their health.

INTRODUCTION

Let's face it, most of us hate exercise. It's boring, hard work and before long we tend to give up, wondering why on earth we started it in the first place. What usually happens then is that an uneasy guilt begins to nag at us, because we know that we really should be making some sort of an effort to get in shape and keep fit. However, filled with the daunting prospect of another gruelling workout, we put it off.

If this scenario sounds at all familiar, this book is good news for you. I have devised a very pleasant and gentle way of moving, stretching and improving your body that you will really enjoy. It is not like traditional exercise or aerobics and it is definitely NOT hard work. It is called YOGACISE and it needs no preparation, and no special clothes, so you are ready to begin right now.

Yogacise is easy and fun to do no matter what your age, shape or condition. It simply involves you moving your body smoothly and slowly to music in a way that will stretch and extend it without you feeling any pain or strain whatsoever. Yet in spite of the mildness of these movements, Yogacise will rapidly slim, firm and condition your entire body and be really relaxing as well. All you will feel is good!

HOW YOGACISE WAS BORN

I have been involved with exercise, dance, fitness, yoga and relaxation professionally for most of my life, so I understand and appreciate very well the value of moving the body as a means of getting and keeping fit. However, I also know that a great many people, myself included, are put off by strenuous exercise because they find it agonising, exhausting and extremely unpleasant to do.

As a professional dancer I had regularly to endure violent exercise sessions during my lengthy training period. I hated them, and I can remember being very depressed at the time because I knew that, even after giving up dancing as a career, I would always want to keep my body fit and in good shape. I assumed that, in order to stay in good condition, I would have to continue forever to put myself through physically tough workouts. Imagine, then, my delight and surprise when, some years later, I was to discover that very gentle movement could actually be far more physically beneficial than violent exercise, giving the lie to the phrase, 'It has to hurt to do you good'. I also discovered how working gently with the body could also bring many mental and emotional benefits. I felt as though a miraculous shift had taken place in my life. Having spent years being cruel to my body, I was now being gentle and kind to it. And it felt wonderful!

Out of this knowledge my own gentle form of yoga was born and it has proved very popular with the public over the past twenty years or so. However, some people who otherwise would be attracted to yoga might be put off because there is a degree of seriousness and discipline needed to practise it. Also, some of the positions and breathing techniques can seem a bit daunting. So, I decided to create an even simpler form of movement that would not require the same dedication, concentration or serious attitude usually associated with yoga, but that would nevertheless still bring wonderful physical and mental benefits. This new way of moving, though still based on yoga, could be done in a much more lighthearted and fun way.

This was to be a system of moving and improving the body that could not possibly daunt anyone. In my experience, people will be able to get and keep fit forever if they can find a way of exercising that is neither physically nor mentally too demanding. This, then, was the aim and, as a result, Yogacise was conceived and born.

WHAT IS YOGACISE?

Yogacise is really a new approach to health and fitness. It is simply a series of continuous body movements that enable virtually anyone to move, stretch and relax their body to music in a slow, rhythmic and very pleasurable way. Yogacise is not only a calming and relaxing way to move the body but, more importantly, it will also quickly bring firmness, fitness, suppleness and strength, even if you have never exercised before.

Compared to most other forms of exercise, Yogacise wil' seem very undemanding. This is because there is no need to 'push' yourself in an attempt to go further and further. 'No sweat!' is how Yogacise can best be described, because you should definitely not perspire or feel exhausted when you do it. With Yogacise, even though the movements are done slowly and smoothly, requiring very little effort on your part, your muscles and joints are nevertheless being thoroughly worked. Both during and after your practice you will feel stretched, refreshed and revitalised. With Yogacise, you will also never be required to hold any positions still or to follow any complicated breathing procedures.

For this book, I have devised thirty-eight Yogacise movements that will move and improve virtually every part of your body from head to toe, and relax you at the same time. The movements are all clearly illustrated with easy-to-follow pictures and instructions beginning on page 21.

CAN ANYBODY DO YOGACISE?

~~~~~~~~~~~~~~

Virtually anyone and everyone can do Yogacise because it is so very simple and requires absolutely no preparation. You can do it even if you have never done any form of exercise before.

It makes no difference whether you are fat or thin, young or old, male or female. Just a few minutes of practice a day is all that you need to feel the rapid improvements that Yogacise will make to your physical and mental fitness and well-being.

There is really only one prerequisite needed to practise Yogacise and that is a desire to get and keep yourself fit in the quickest, easiest and most pleasant way possible.

IS YOGACISE SAFE?

~~~~~~~~~~~~~~

Yogacise has been designed to be absolutely safe for anyone, no matter what their age or state of physical fitness. This means that Yogacise can be done in the confidence of knowing that you won't do yourself any harm. This applies even if you regard yourself as being totally out of shape and unfit. It also means that you can do as much or as little Yogacise as you like.

The reason that Yogacise is so safe is that the movements are performed gently to music in a continuous, dance-like, fluid way and you are constantly aware of what is happening to your body. If you were to feel any sensations of pain, strain or tightness anywhere, you should automatically stop because, with this form of exercise, absolutely NO PAIN OR STRAIN SHOULD EVER BE FELT. With Yogacise, you will simply feel that you are pleasantly stretching and then relaxing your body.

SOME CAUTIONS

Yogacise is absolutely safe because it is probably the mildest form of exercise around. However, if you suspect that you may be suffering from a medical condition that could be exacerbated by doing Yogacise, show this book to your doctor and get his or her approval before you begin.

PREGNANCY CAUTION

Yogacise is an ideal way to keep fit during pregnancy, and certain movements are particularly beneficial. Other Yogacise movements should, however, be avoided during pregnancy. You will find information on how to practise Yogacise safely when pregnant on page 90.

IS THERE AN AGE LIMIT
FOR YOGACISE?

Absolutely not! You can practise Yogacise whether you are a tiny tot or approaching your one-hundredth birthday.

In fact, the safety of Yogacise means that it is a particularly good way for senior citizens to move their bodies and keep them strong, supple, slim and fit, and to enjoy themselves at the same time. The older we get the more important it is to keep the body strong and flexible, but many elderly people are put off doing conventional exercises because, quite rightly, they do not want to leap around getting exhausted or risk injuring themselves. They will find that Yogacise is ideal in this respect, because it will bring all the benefits of exercise without any danger.

Children also love to bend and move their bodies, and Yogacise gives them an alternative to the more boisterous sports and physical education usually taught in schools. It is also a fact that some children feel a sense of inadequacy if they are not very good at PE, which can cause them to reject all forms of exercise for life. This means that their general fitness is neglected and can lead to all sorts of health problems later on. Because Yogacise is easy and fun for children to do, it can become very popular with them. So much so that they adopt Yogacise as a means of keeping fit for life.

So if you have children, try doing Yogacise with them. It can be a treat for the whole family.

WHAT ARE THE PHYSICAL BENEFITS
OF YOGACISE?

In order to get and stay in good condition, we all need to move our bodies much more than our rather sedentary lifestyles allow us to do these days. This also applies to people who tend to rush around a lot in the course of their lives, because although they might be using up a lot of energy, they may not necessarily be receiving the right sort of exercise to get and keep their bodies fit.

Good health and fitness come from having a strong, supple, flexible body. To achieve this we need gently but thoroughly to stretch the body, and work all of the muscles and joints regularly. We also need to keep our lungs working well so that we take in the maximum amount of air and oxygen when we breathe. The practice of Yogacise will enable you to do all this and much more because it works virtually every single part of your body.

Here are some of the physical benefits of Yogacise. It will:

- slim and firm your body, eliminating any excess weight
- slim and firm specific areas of your body such as the tummy, thighs, hips, bottom, waist, upper arms and neck
- increase the strength and mobility of your shoulders, arms, hands, wrists and fingers
- increase the strength and mobility of your legs, feet, ankles and toes
- greatly improve the suppleness and strength of your back
- improve posture, deportment and balance
- remove tension
- relax you completely
- ease backache caused by stiffness
- ease tension and stiffness from your shoulders and neck
- improve circulation throughout your body
- increase your level of energy and vitality
- eliminate stress headaches
- promote deeper and improved breathing
- improve your sense of rhythm
- improve the quality of your sleep
- reduce fatigue generally
- help to alleviate the physical symptoms of PMT.

WHAT ARE THE MENTAL AND EMOTIONAL BENEFITS OF YOGACISE?

Our bodies, our minds and our emotions all need time off to relax, but most of us find this extremely difficult to achieve. People often say to me, 'I try so hard to relax but I just can't do it.' The truth is that you can't MAKE yourself relax; you have to ALLOW yourself to relax completely. The first necessity of relaxation is the release of any tension and stress from the body. Only then can your mind and your emotions follow suit. Yogacise will enable you to do this because, as you are going through the movements, you will also be breathing in a particular way that enables you automatically to let go of all the tension inside you, both physical and mental. And this complete relaxation will happen without you having to make any conscious effort to bring it about.

Relaxation, and a sense of peace and calm, is one of the major mental and emotional benefits of Yogacise, but it can also bring other benefits. It can alleviate depression, listlessness and apathy, relieve strain generally from your life, and increase your mental and emotional awareness and sensitivity. It can also improve your confidence, and greatly ease the mental and emotional problems of PMT.

WHEN SHOULD I DO YOGACISE
AND FOR HOW LONG?

You can practise Yogacise for as little or as much time as you like. If you only have five minutes a day to spare, even that would be enough to get and keep you in good shape. This means that no matter how busy your life, you will be able to fit some Yogacise into it. Should you have a little more time, however, it is fine to extend your practice to ten or fifteen minutes a day.

One thing that you will quickly discover when you begin to practise Yogacise, is that it feels so good that it is highly likely you will want to spend longer and longer doing it. And, of course, the more Yogacise you do, the more benefit you will get out of it.

You may prefer not to do Yogacise every day, and it is fine to do it on, say, alternate days of the week. You may want to restrict your sessions to perhaps only two or three a week and that is all right too. How much Yogacise you do and how often is entirely up to you. Just tailor your practice to suit your life.

Yogacise can be practised at any time of the day, except perhaps after a heavy meal, when it could feel a little uncomfortable.

WHERE SHOULD I DO YOGACISE?

You can do Yogacise virtually anywhere. All you need is enough space around you so that you can stretch up and out with your arms without hitting the furniture. You also need to have sufficient space in which to lie comfortably on the floor.

Yogacise can be practised in any room at home or in the garden, or for that matter on the beach.

WHAT SHOULD I WEAR TO PRACTISE?

The beauty of Yogacise is that there are no special clothes that you have to buy or wear in order to practise. You can forget the idea of having to change into exercise clothes such as a leotard or tracksuit and simply wear your normal, everyday clothes. Obviously, it would be better not to have anything on that is too uncomfortable as it would distract you. Also, if you are wearing something that is tight around the waist, just loosen it a little or undo it.

For comfort, you may also decide that you want to kick your shoes off, but you don't have to.

WHY MUSIC?

I have added the dimension of music to Yogacise because it enhances practice, increasing both its physical and mental benefits. This happens because the body tends to flow more smoothly when one is moving to music, and it is by moving in this way that the body will become rapidly supple and strong. Music also has the effect of cutting out any external noise and enabling you to create exactly the sort of atmosphere that you want. Also, most people get an enormous amount of pleasure when moving their bodies to music because they enjoy the sense of dance that it gives them.

The type of music that you choose is entirely up to you, but I find that most people like to do Yogacise to something gentle and relaxing. Use a record, a tape or a CD, or even the radio if you prefer.

It is not, of course, absolutely essential to do Yogacise to music. In fact, some people find that it is wonderfully peaceful to practise in total silence.

ON YOUR OWN OR IN A GROUP?

Most people will probably practise Yogacise on their own, but there is absolutely no reason why you should not do it in a group if you prefer. Since the Yogacise movements require very little concentration, you need not worry that other people will be disturbing you. It can also be great fun to do Yogacise with other members of your family.

YOGACISE FOR LIFE

Most forms of keep fit or exercise are short-lived affairs. We begin them full of enthusiasm and good intentions, only to give them up again after only a few weeks or months. The reason for this is that most exercise regimes demand too much of us either in the way of time or effort. I believe that in order for exercise to have a really permanent place in our lives, it has to be three things. First, it has to be genuinely easy and pleasant to do. Secondly, it has to be effective and, thirdly, it should not cause disruption or inconvenience. Yogacise satisfies these three criteria.

Once Yogacise is established in your life you may find, as do many of my students, that you actually feel resentful if, for any reason, you are prevented from doing your regular practice.

Yogacise is an ideal way of getting fit and then keeping yourself in good condition for life. It could become one of your most valuable habits.

HOW TO USE THIS BOOK

In the practice section beginning on page 21, you will find thirty-eight Yogacise movements. Each movement is clearly illustrated with step-by-step pictures and instructions. With each movement you will also find details about its particular benefits, both physical and mental.

The Yogacise movements can either be done individually or linked together into short routines. You can select the movements for your practice sessions yourself or, if you prefer, you can follow the routines that I have prepared which begin on page 87. These routines are for five, ten and fifteen minutes and have been specially designed to ensure that virtually every part of your body is worked on.

How many and which movements you do in your practice sessions will depend upon your time and the benefits that you desire. Also, you will probably find that certain movements become particular favourites. Do as many or as few Yogacise movements as you like.

There are specific movements in the book that can be used very effectively to help to slim and firm certain areas of the body. There are also particular movements that will help to alleviate some physical, mental or emotional conditions. By referring to the glossary on pages 91 to 95, you will discover which movements are recommended for your particular problem.

There is a special section on Yogacise and pregnancy on page 90.

An important point you should always remember when practising Yogacise is that you should not feel any pain or strain. If you do, this is a good indication that you are making too much effort. Unlike conventional exercise there is no need to think of 'working your body' or of getting hot and exhausted. I feel that in order to be fit for life rather than for the next aerobics class, you need to be able gently to firm, slim and condition your body from head to toe, and this is what Yogacise does. Unlike more conventional exercise, however, Yogacise accomplishes its aim in an essentially very safe, undemanding and enjoyable way.

Yogacise is extremely pleasant to do and from your first practice session you should begin to feel good both physically and mentally. This would even be the case if your session lasted for only five minutes.

Now you are ready to begin, so turn to the practice section, put on some nice music and get started!

PRACTICE INTRODUCTION

When practising Yogacise, remember not to rush the movements but to move smoothly to the music. Use four beats of music to go into the position and four beats to come out of it. If you are practising without music, simply count four to yourself at approximately one-second intervals.

As you regularly practise Yogacise, you will find that without really trying, you are automatically able to go further as your body stretches and strengthens. As a guide, I have therefore included some pictures of more advanced positions, but I do not want you to try to get into these positions prematurely. Remember that with Yogacise there is no pushing or forcing, so just work gently and you will progress at the right pace.

The simple breathing instructions for Yogacise are given in the appropriate photo captions. You will find that the breathing feels completely natural because it is merely an exaggeration of the way that you would breathe automatically. If, however, you find any problems in trying to incorporate the breathing instructions, then it is absolutely fine to practise without using them.

STANDING BREATH

The Standing Breath strengthens the back, shoulders and arms. It works the lungs, improving breathing generally, and it is also very relaxing.

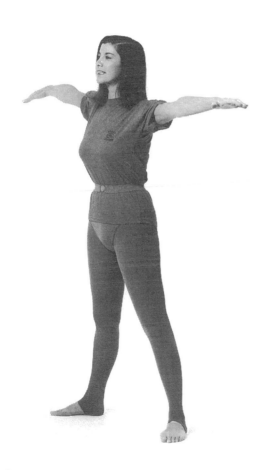 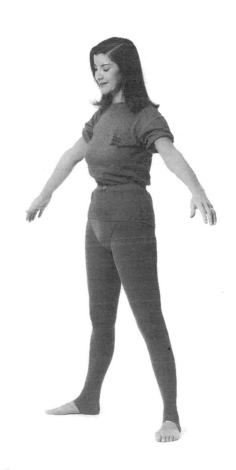

1 Stand legs apart and inhale as you raise the arms to shoulder level for 4 beats.

2 Lower the arms as you breathe out for 4 beats.
Repeat movement 8 times.

Standing Movements

STANDING REACH-UP

SINGLE ARM

The Reach-Up stretches and firms the sides of the body. It also strengthens the back, shoulders, arms and hands.

There are two versions of this movement. The first is to reach up and then relax your arm down, as shown in photo 2. The second version is to extend your arm out to the side as you bring it down, as shown in photos 3 and 4. Practise both versions as indicated.

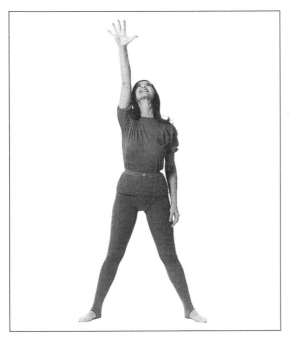 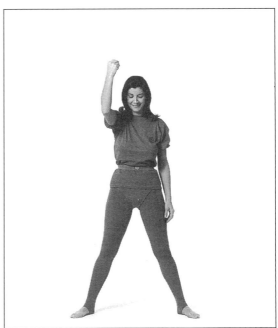

1 Stand with legs apart and stretch one arm up as high as you can for 4 beats, breathing in at the same time.

2 Relax the arm down as you breathe out for 4 beats.
Repeat the movement 4 times, then do it with the other arm. (Repeat again, 4 times with each arm, when you are stronger.)

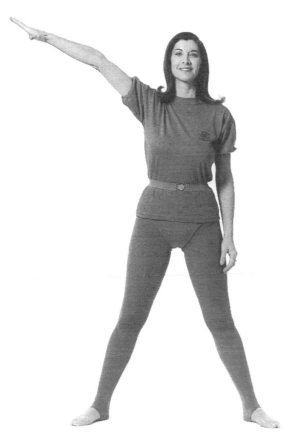

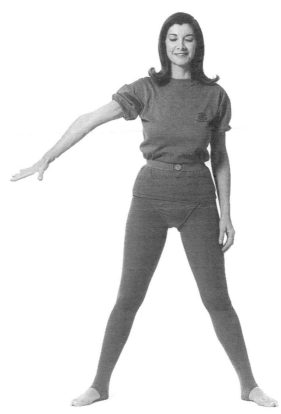

③ Stretch arm up as shown in photo 1, but extend it out to the sides on the way down.

④ Continue lowering the arm to the side. Repeat movement 4 times with each arm. (Repeat again, 4 times with each arm, when you are stronger.)

STANDING REACH-UP

BOTH ARMS

The Reach-Up with both arms stretches the back and the sides, and flattens and firms the stomach. It also strengthens the back, shoulders, arms and hands.

As with the single arm Reach-Up, there are two version of this movement. In the first you reach up and then relax your arms down, as shown in photo 2. In the second version you stretch your arms out to the sides as they come down, as shown in photos 3 and 4. Practise both versions as indicated.

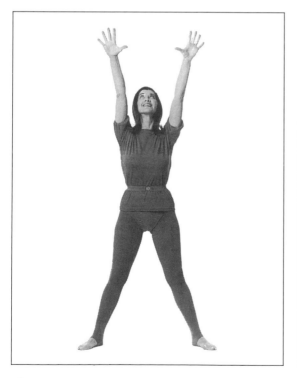

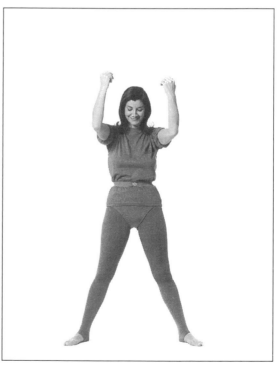

1   Stand with legs apart and stretch both arms as high as you can for 4 beats, breathing in at the same time.

2   Relax the arms down as you breathe out for 4 beats.
Repeat movement 8 times.

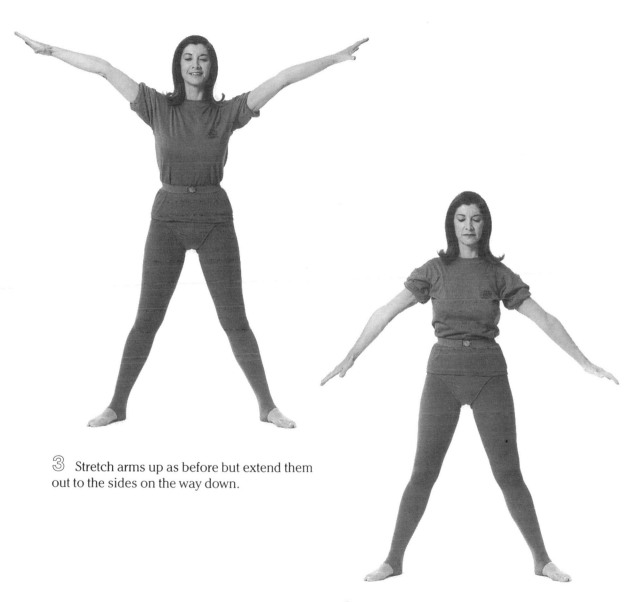

③ Stretch arms up as before but extend them out to the sides on the way down.

④ Continue lowering the arms to the sides. Repeat movement 8 times.

SIDE SLIDE

The Side Slide stretches the sides of the body and slims the waist. It also strengthens the back and improves balance.

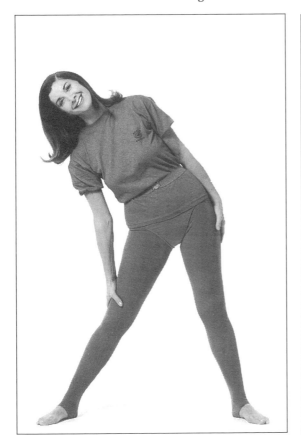 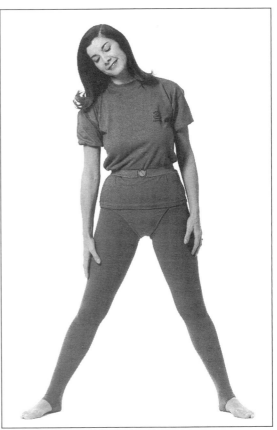

1 Bend over to the right side, sliding your right hand down the leg and the left hand up the left leg for 4 beats, exhaling as you go.

2 Straighten up for 4 beats, breathing in. Then exhale as you repeat over to the other side. Repeat movement 4 times on alternate sides, 8 times in all. (Repeat again, 4 times on each side, when you are stronger.)

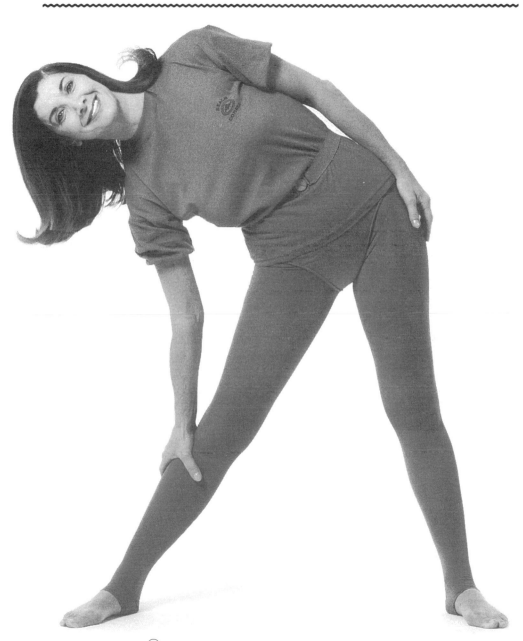

③ In time you will be able to bend further over to each side.

TRIANGLE

The Triangle stretches, slims, and firms the sides and the upper arms. It also strengthens the back, shoulders and legs, and improves balance and co-ordination.

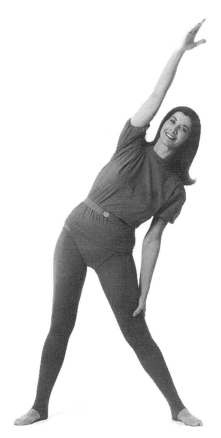

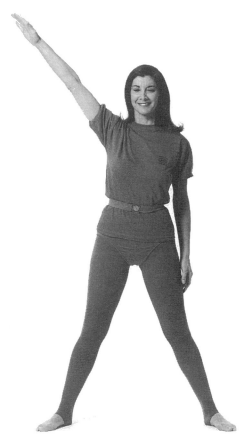

1 Stand with legs apart and bend over to one side for 4 beats, taking hold of the leg and raising the other arm over your head. Breathe out as you go over.

2 Straighten up for 4 beats, breathing in so you are ready to repeat on the other side. Repeat movement 4 times on alternate sides, 8 times in all. (Repeat again, 4 times on each side, when you are stronger.)

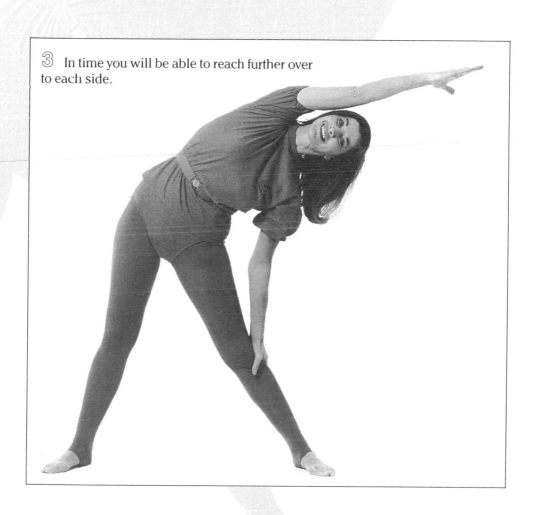

③ In time you will be able to reach further over to each side.

FORWARD BEND

This movement stretches and strengthens the back and neck, and relaxes the neck, shoulders, arms and hands. It also increases the blood flow into the head and face, which not only improves the complexion, but also has a generally revitalising effect.

Try not to push your body over. Simply let it relax over as shown in photo 1.

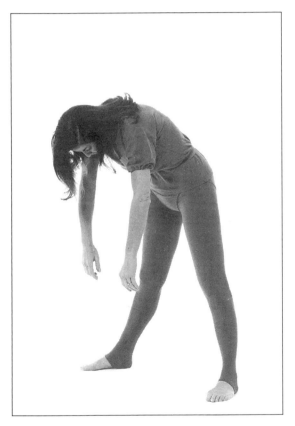

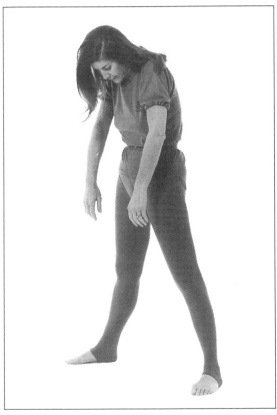

1 Exhale as you relax your body over for 4 beats.

2 Inhale as you uncoil your back for 4 beats, until you are upright again.
Repeat movement 8 times.

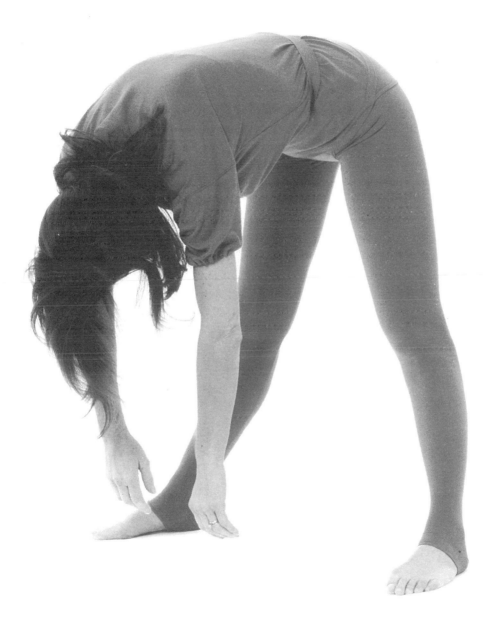

③ In time you will be able to relax further over.

SQUAT

The Squat strengthens the legs, knees and back and greatly improves balance. It will also slim, firm and tone the thighs. Try the basic movement first, as in photo 1, and once you feel comfortable with that, you may like to try the variations shown in photos 2, 3 and 4. Practice of these variations will also strengthen the shoulders and the arms.

To begin with only bend your knees a little. As your muscles strengthen, you will find that you can naturally go further.

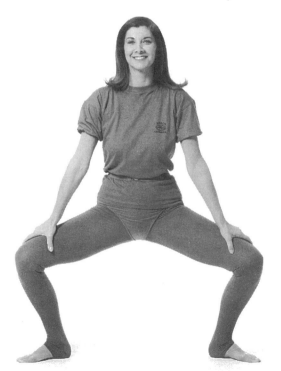

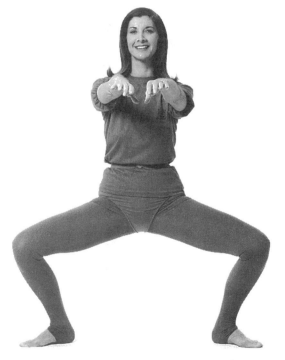

1 Bend both knees outwards, holding the thighs if desired, and breathing out for 4 beats. Then straighten up, breathing in for 4 beats. Repeat 8 times.

2 Bring the arms up in front of you as you bend the knees. Repeat 8 times.

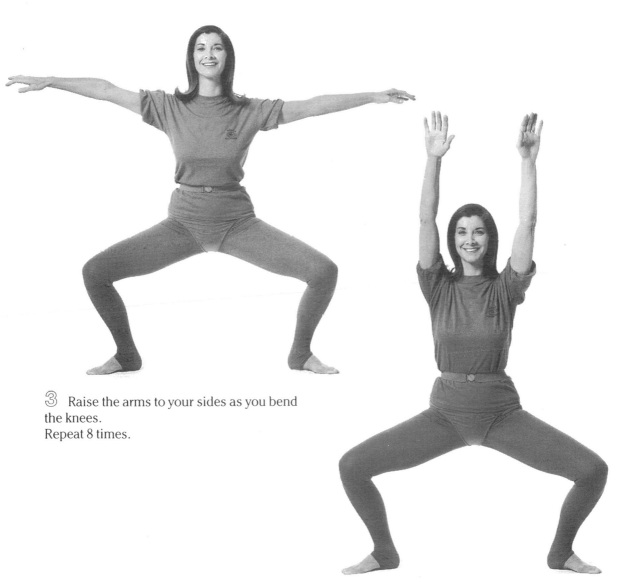

3 Raise the arms to your sides as you bend the knees.
Repeat 8 times.

4 Raise the arms right above your head as you bend the knees.
Repeat 8 times.

KNEELING REACH-UP

This movement firms and slims the thighs, waist and stomach. It also strengthens and stretches the back, shoulders, arms and hands.

Kneeling Movements

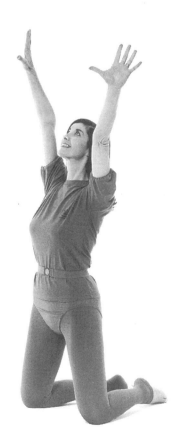
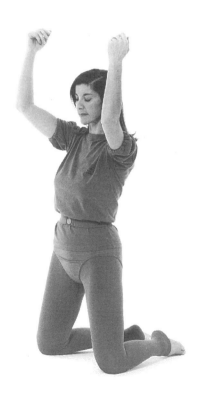

1   Kneel with legs apart and stretch up with both arms, breathing in for 4 beats.

2   Relax arms down as you breathe out for 4 beats.
Repeat 8 times.

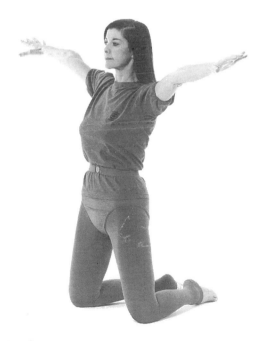

4 The Reach-Up can also be done sitting back on the heels if the position is comfortable for you.

3 Do the Reach-Up again, but this time stretch the arms out on the way down.
Repeat 8 times.

SIT DOWN

This movement firms and slims the buttocks, stomach and thighs, as well as strengthening the back, shoulders and arms.

In order to get the benefit from this movement, it is important that you DO NOT SIT RIGHT DOWN when you do it. Just come down a little way, as shown in photo 1.

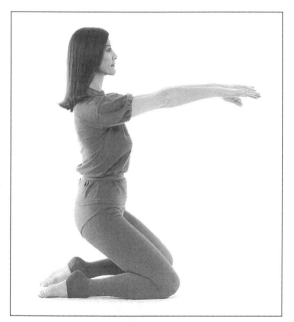

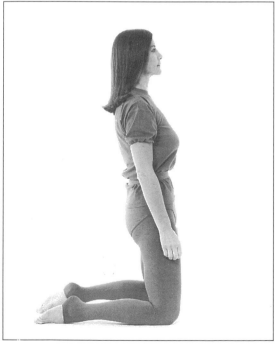

1 Bring your bottom down towards the floor, raising your arms at the same time and exhaling for 4 beats.

2 Inhale as you straighten up, tightening the buttocks and lowering your arms for 4 beats. Repeat 8 times.

KNEELING BACK WAVE

The Back Wave really increases suppleness and strength throughout the back and neck and is very relaxing to do.

I call this the Back Wave because you should feel a little bit as though your back is making a wave-like movement as you straighten it up.

If you find this position uncomfortable, try the seated Back Wave on page 50.

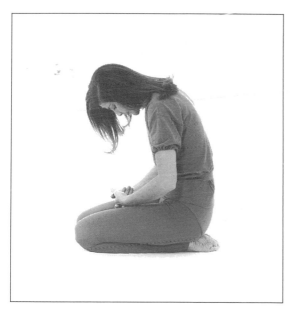

1 Sit on your heels with your back, shoulders, head, arms and hands relaxed.

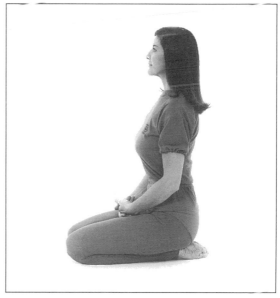

2 Breathe in as you straighten your back and head for 4 beats.
Exhale as you relax back into position 1 for 4 beats. Repeat 8 times.

UNCOIL

The Uncoil greatly strengthens the back and increases suppleness and flexibility. It also helps to flatten the stomach.

The movement is called the Uncoil because that is literally what the back does as it straightens up. To help you to do this properly, try to keep the back rounded as you bring it up and raise your head last.

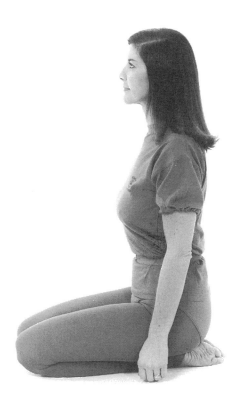

1 Sit on your heels with your arms at your sides.

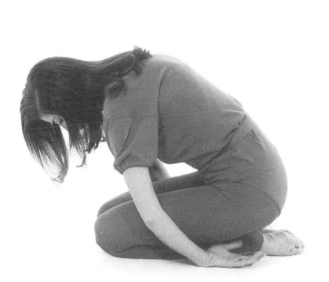

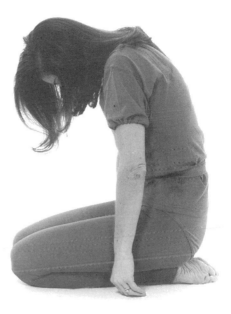

2   Relax forward for 4 beats, breathing out.

3   Uncoil your back, breathing in for 4 beats. Repeat 8 times.

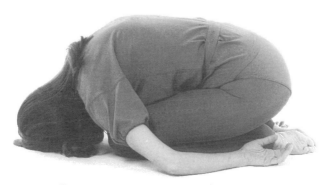

4   In time you will be able to go further forward.

CAT

The Yogacise Cat brings many benefits. It greatly strengthens the back, increasing suppleness and flexibility. It firms and slims the buttocks, hips, waist and stomach. It also strengthens the neck, shoulders, arms and wrists and works out any stiffness and tension in the neck and shoulder area.

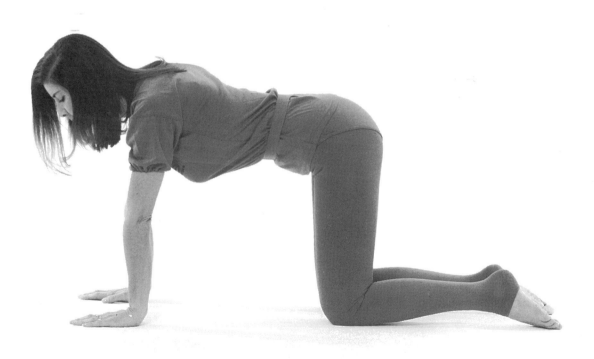

1 Start from this position.

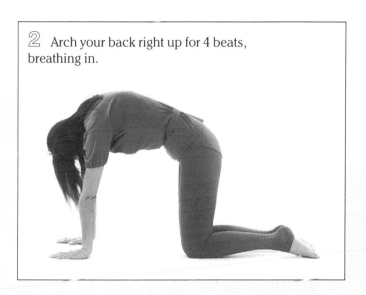

2 Arch your back right up for 4 beats, breathing in.

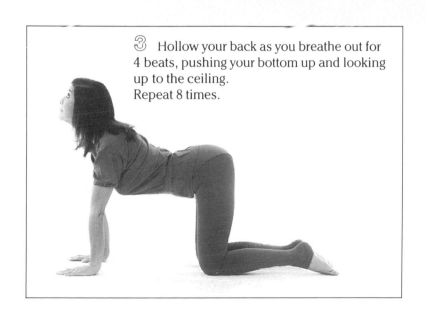

3 Hollow your back as you breathe out for 4 beats, pushing your bottom up and looking up to the ceiling.
Repeat 8 times.

'V'

This movement stretches the back and the legs, and strengthens the toes, ankles, shoulders, arms and wrists. It also slims and firms the thighs. An additional benefit of the 'V' is that it improves the complexion and is refreshing and revitalising.

Push your body up into a 'V' shape when you do it.

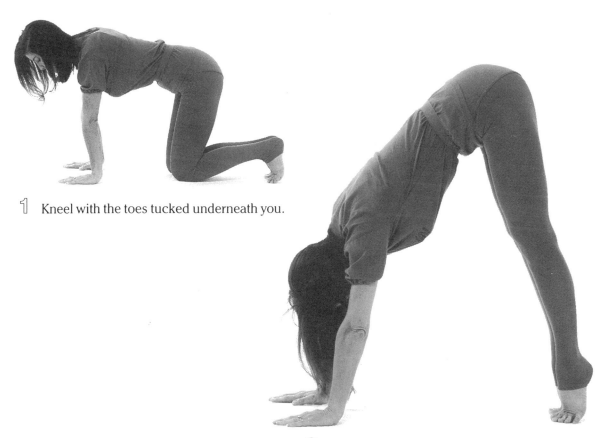

1 Kneel with the toes tucked underneath you.

2 Push up for 4 beats, breathing in.

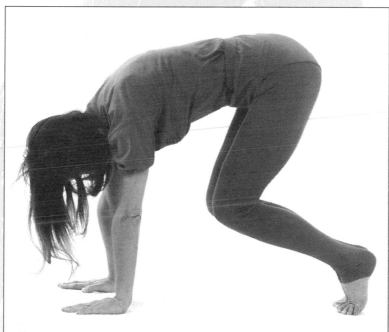

③ Bend the knees smoothly, breathing out, for 4 beats. Repeat 4 times. (Repeat again 4 times when you are stronger.)

SEATED REACH-UP

The seated Reach-Up is not only valuable for establishing and then maintaining the strength of the back, shoulders and arms, but it also strengthens, firms and slims the legs and stretches the sides.

Do the first version with the legs together, as in photo 1, and when your strength has increased a little, you may like to try the other versions.

1 Reach up and inhale for 4 beats.
Exhale and let the arms relax down for 4 beats.
Repeat 8 times.

Repeat a further 8 times, stretching the arms out to the sides as they come down.

2 Sit with the legs apart.
Then follow the instructions as for photo 1.

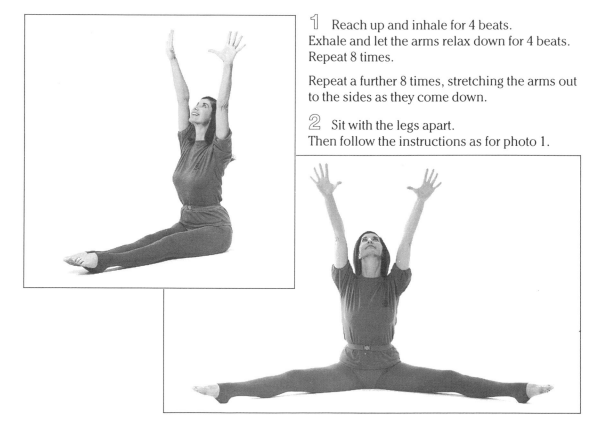

Sitting Movements

44

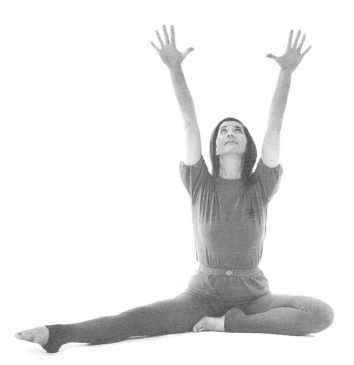

3 Bend one knee.
Then follow the instructions as for photo 1.

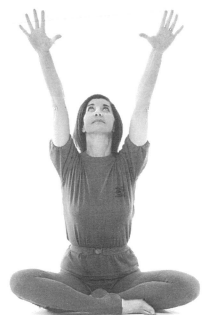

4 Sit with the legs crossed.
Then follow the instructions as for photo 1.

HEAD TO KNEES

This movement stretches and conditions the neck and back, and works out any stiffness and tension in that area.

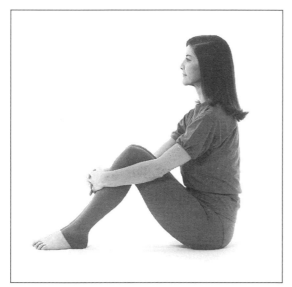

1 Interlock the fingers and loop the hands around the knees.

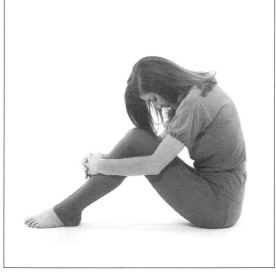

2 Bring your head down towards your knees, exhaling for 4 beats.
Inhale as you return to position 1 for 4 beats.
Repeat 8 times.

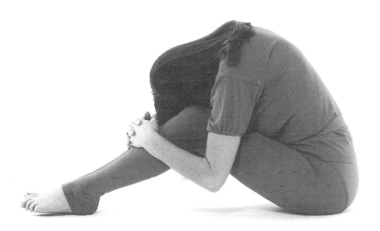

③ After practising for a while, lower your knees a little so that your back bends over further.

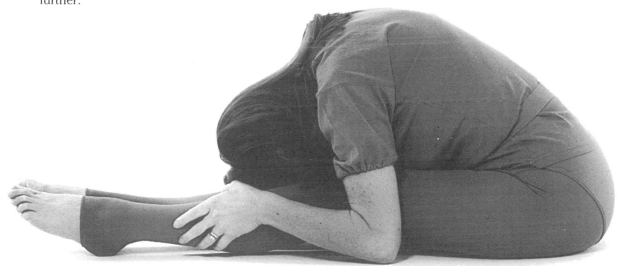

④ In time you may be able to bend over this far with your legs completely straight.

SHOULDER TWIST

The Shoulder Twist slims and firms the waist, and strengthens the back, shoulders, neck and arms.

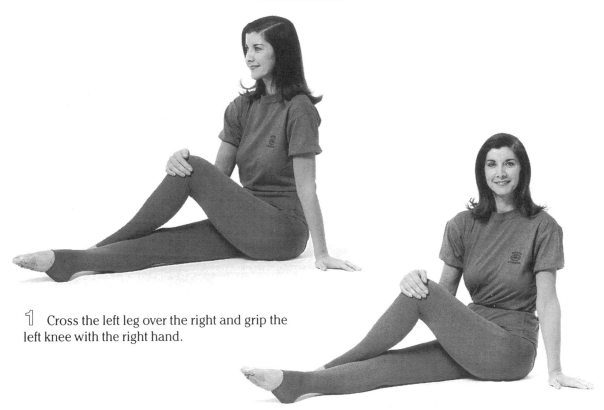

1 Cross the left leg over the right and grip the left knee with the right hand.

2 Inhale as you twist your shoulders to the left for 4 beats.
Exhale as you return your shoulders to the front for 4 beats.
Repeat 4 times, then change sides. (Repeat again, 4 times on both sides, when you are stronger.)

③ In time you will be able to twist round further.

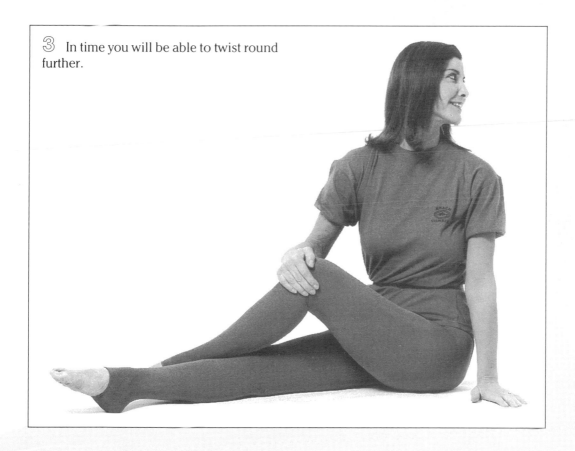

SEATED BACK WAVE

The seated Back Wave increases strength and suppleness throughout the back and neck. It also strengthens the shoulders, arms and wrists.

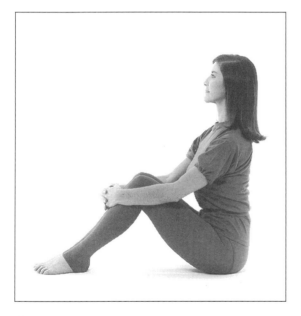

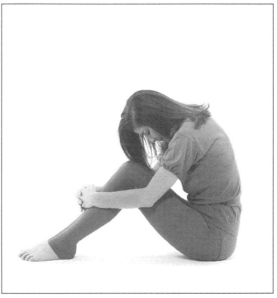

1 Sit with the hands interlocked around the knees.
Breathe in and pull your back up as straight as you can for 4 beats.

2 Exhale, and relax your back and head over for 4 beats.
Repeat 8 times.

SHOULDER ROTATIONS

This movement works out any stiffness and tension from the shoulders, neck and the top of the back. It is very good for both relaxing and removing stress.

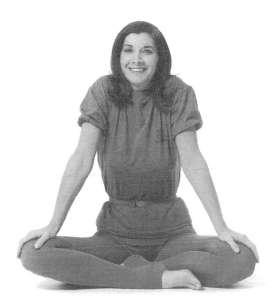

1 Inhale as you take the shoulders forward and up for 4 beats.

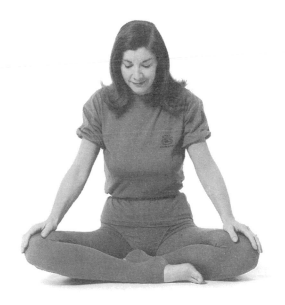

2 Exhale as the shoulders relax back and down for 4 beats.
Repeat 8 times.

ARM CIRCLING

This movement greatly strengthens the arms, shoulders and back.

Use only one beat of music for each arm rotation and do four rotations forwards and four backwards. Then repeat. Breathe normally when doing the movement.

1 Make fists of the hands and, keeping the arms straight, rotate the arms forward 4 times. Then rotate the arms backwards 4 times. Repeat forward and backward rotations again.

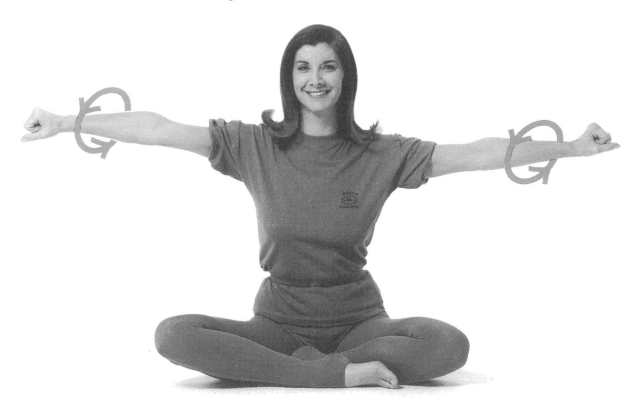

ELBOW BENDS

Elbow Bends work the elbow joints to keep them healthy. This movement also strengthens the shoulders and arms.

Just breathe normally when doing this movement.

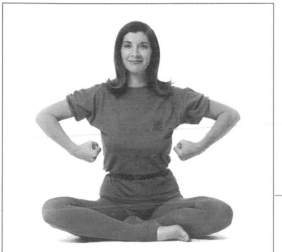

1 Make fists of the hands and bend them in for 1 beat of the music.

2 Extend the arms out to the sides for 1 beat of the music.
Repeat 8 times.

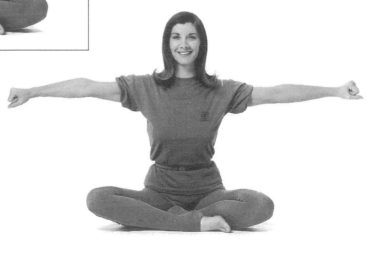

HEAD ROLL

The Head Roll is a wonderfully relaxing movement to do. It stretches the neck and works out stiffness and tension from the neck and the top of the back.

Just breathe normally when you do it and use four beats of music for each rotation.

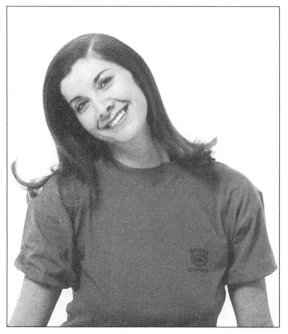

1 Roll your head gently around to the right.

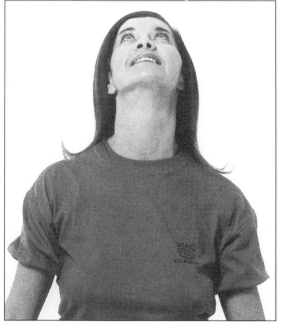

2 Roll your head to the back.

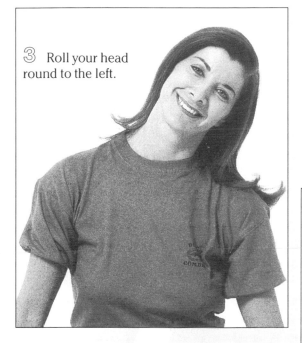

3 Roll your head round to the left.

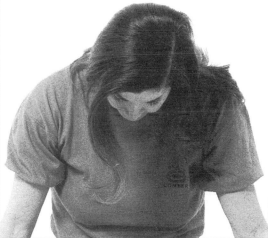

4 Roll your head round to the front. Repeat thc movement 4 times and then do it 4 times in the opposite direction. Repeat again, 4 times in each direction.

EYE ROTATIONS

This movement works the eye muscles to keep them healthy.

Just breathe normally when you do it and use four beats of music for each complete
eye rotation.

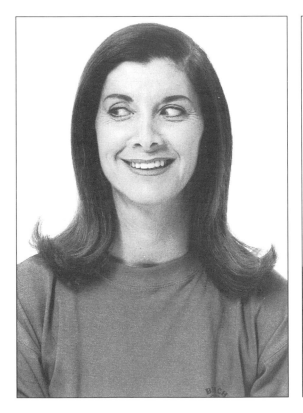

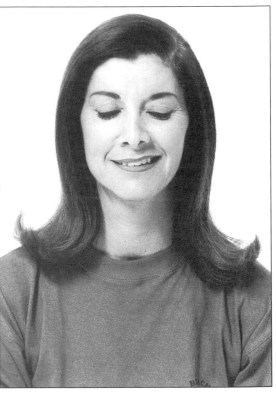

1 Roll your eyes to the right.

2 Roll your eyes down.

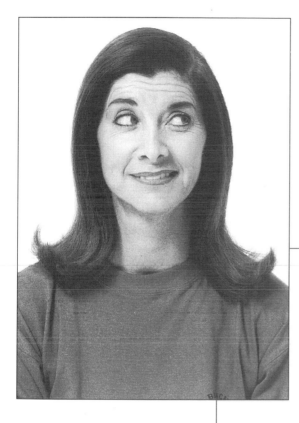

③ Roll your eyes to the left.

④ Roll your eyes up.
Repeat 4 rotations.
Then do the same in the
opposite direction.

FINGER SPREAD

This movement works the muscles of the palms of the hands and the fingers, and strengthens the arms. It also releases tension and stress generally.

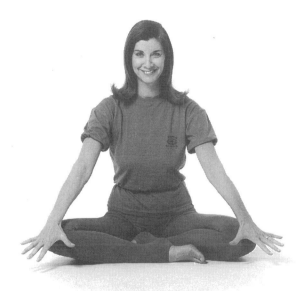

1 Straighten the arms and spread the fingers as wide as you can for 4 beats, breathing in.

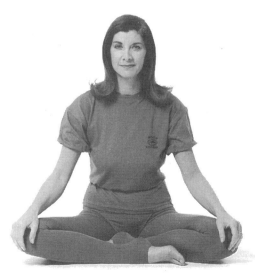

2 Relax your hands for 4 beats, breathing out. Repeat 8 times.

FISTS

This movement works the muscles of the palms of the hands, the fingers and the thumbs. It also strengthens the arms and, as with the Yogacise Finger Spread, releases tension and stress generally.

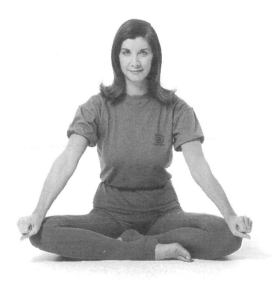

1 Straighten the elbows and make tight fists of the hands for 4 beats, breathing in.

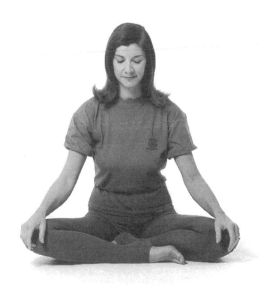

2 Relax your hands for 4 beats, breathing out. Repeat 8 times.

FINGER PULLS

This movement strengthens the finger joints and also the top of the back, shoulders, arms and wrists. It also develops the chest muscles.

Grip as much of each finger as you can, but don't pull it roughly.

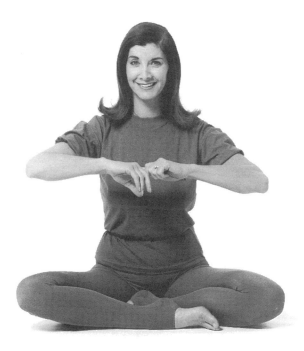

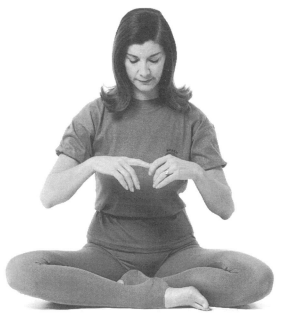

1 Breathe in as you steadily pull one of your fingers for 4 beats.

2 Exhale for 4 beats, as you relax your grip. Continue with all the fingers of one hand, and then repeat with the other hand.

FOOT WORK

This movement will strengthen the muscles and joints of the feet and toes, and slim the ankles. It will also strengthen and firm the legs.

Just breathe normally when doing it.

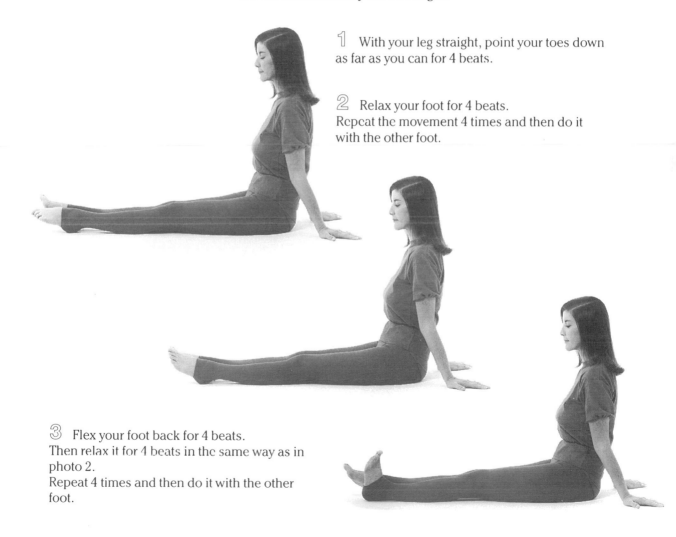

1 With your leg straight, point your toes down as far as you can for 4 beats.

2 Relax your foot for 4 beats.
Repeat the movement 4 times and then do it with the other foot.

3 Flex your foot back for 4 beats.
Then relax it for 4 beats in the same way as in photo 2.
Repeat 4 times and then do it with the other foot.

61

LYING BREATH

This movement will improve breathing generally. It also gives the body a gentle overall stretch.

Lying Movements

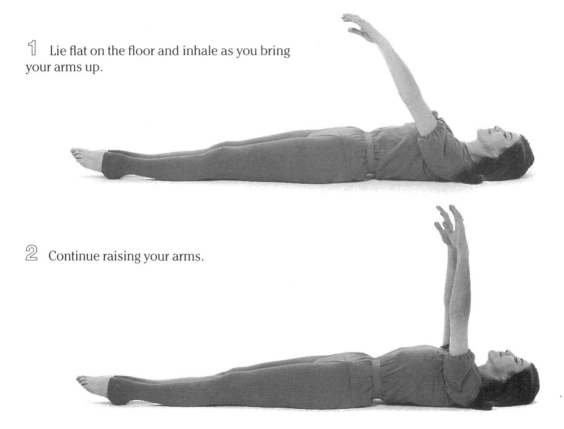

1 Lie flat on the floor and inhale as you bring your arms up.

2 Continue raising your arms.

③ Take 4 beats in total to bring your arms right above your head and on to the floor.

④ Exhale as you bring your arms down again for 4 beats.
Repeat 8 times.

STRETCH

The Stretch gives the body a really thorough stretch from head to toe, firming and strengthening it. It also improves the breathing generally, removes stress and is very relaxing.

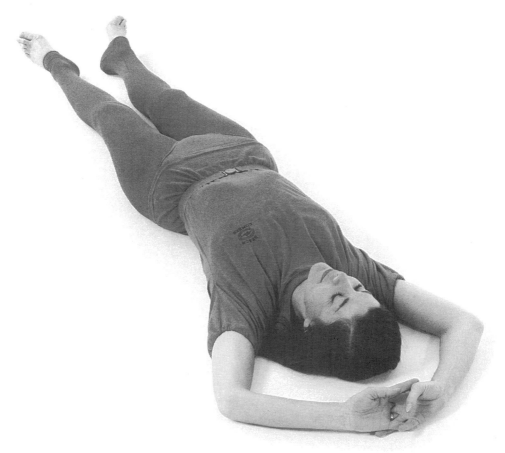

1 Lie flat on the floor and interlock the fingers.

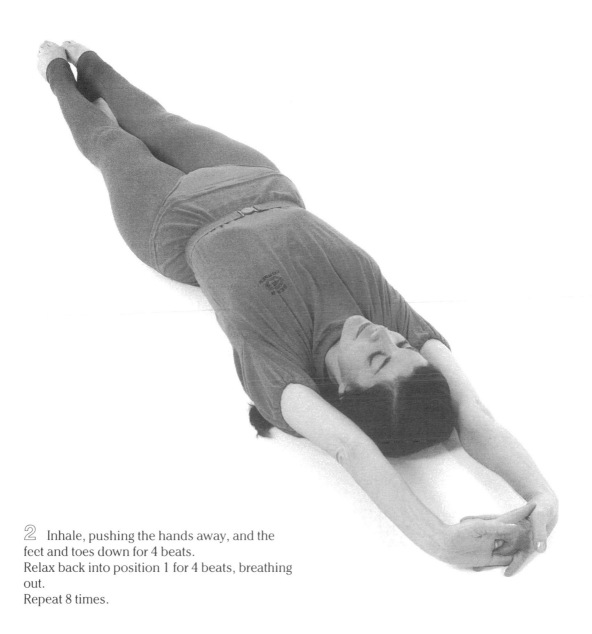

2 Inhale, pushing the hands away, and the feet and toes down for 4 beats.
Relax back into position 1 for 4 beats, breathing out.
Repeat 8 times.

COBRA

This movement greatly strengthens the back, increasing suppleness and flexibility.
It also strengthens the neck, shoulders, arms and wrists, and works out any stiffness
or tension in the neck and the top of the back.

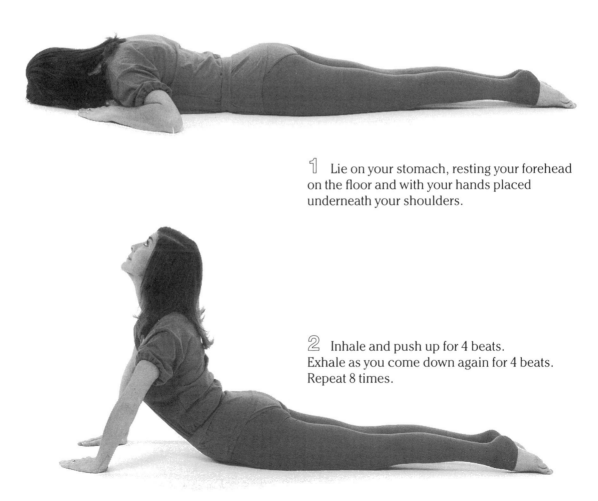

1 Lie on your stomach, resting your forehead
on the floor and with your hands placed
underneath your shoulders.

2 Inhale and push up for 4 beats.
Exhale as you come down again for 4 beats.
Repeat 8 times.

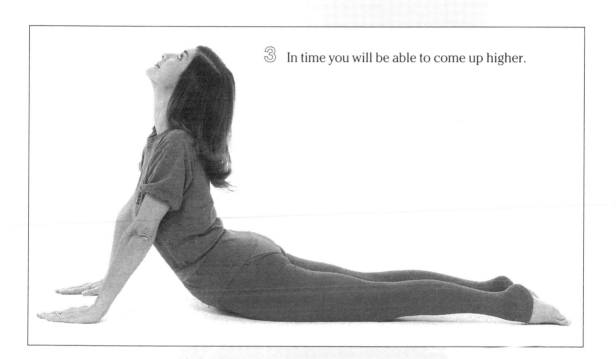

③ In time you will be able to come up higher.

COIL

The Coil stretches the back and the neck, making them strong and flexible. It also strengthens the shoulders, arms, wrists and fingers, and works out any stiffness and tension from the neck area.

1 Lie on your back and interlock your fingers around your bent knees.

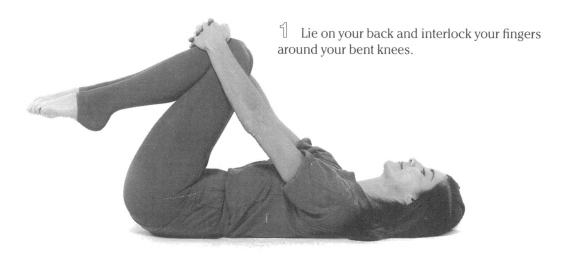

2 Exhale as you bring your head up to your knees for 4 beats.
Inhale as you return to position 1 for 4 beats.
Repeat 8 times.

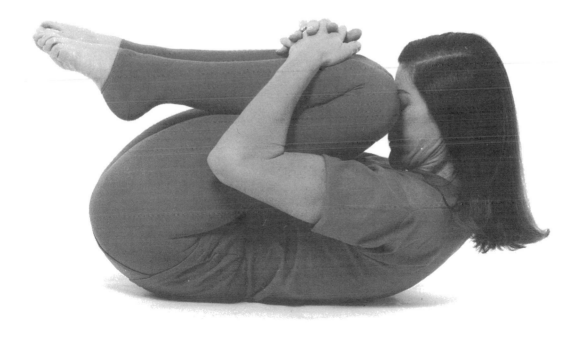

③ In time you will be able to go further.

FISH

The Fish improves strength and suppleness throughout the back. It also strengthens the neck, shoulders and arms, and backward tilting of the head improves the complexion.

The Fish has a wonderfully relaxing effect, especially if you do it with your eyes closed.

(*Note*: You may like to place a silky scarf underneath your head before you start as this will help your head to slide smoothly.)

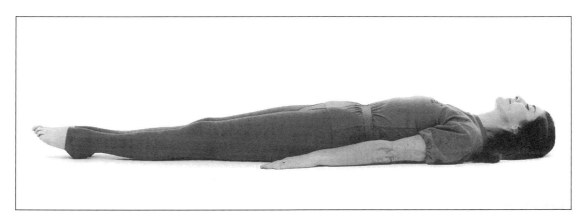

1 Lie on your back.

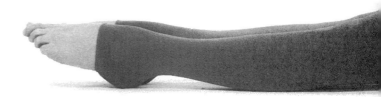

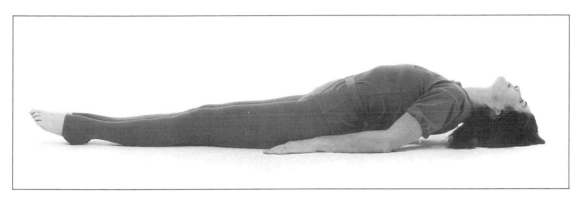

2   Inhale and push down on the floor as you arch your back upwards and tilt your head back, for 4 beats.
Exhale, as your head slides back and you return to position 1 for 4 beats.
Repeat 8 times.

3   In time you will be able to arch your back higher.

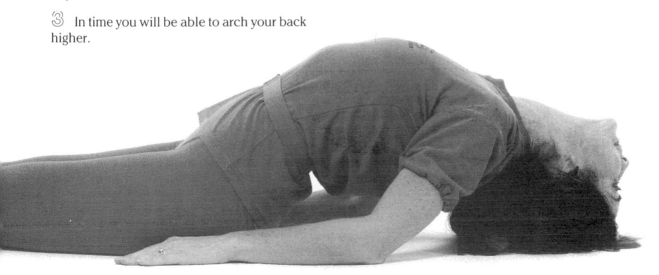

HIP PUSH

This movement strengthens the centre of the back, and firms and slims the thighs and buttocks.

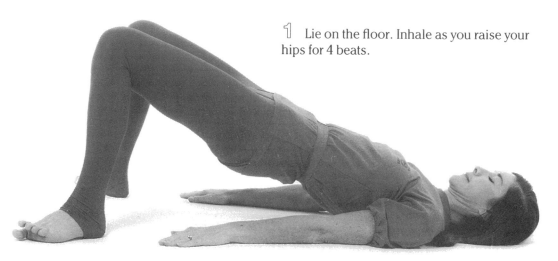

1 Lie on the floor. Inhale as you raise your hips for 4 beats.

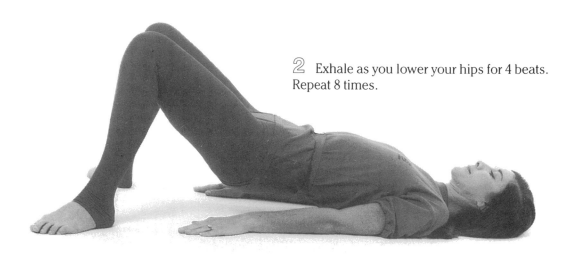

2 Exhale as you lower your hips for 4 beats. Repeat 8 times.

③ In time you will be able to raise your hips higher.

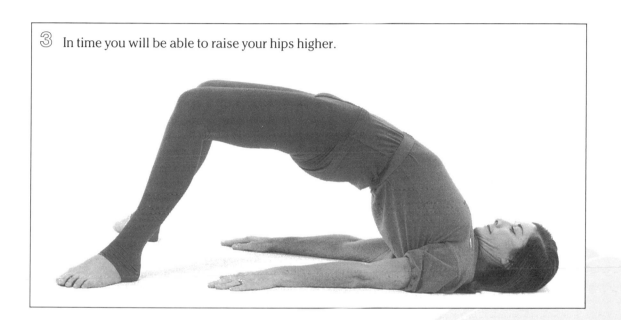

LEG WORK

SINGLE LEG

Leg Work strengthens the muscles and joints of the legs, feet and toes, and slims and firms the thighs and calves.

Just breathe normally when doing this movement.

1 Lie on the floor with your legs together.

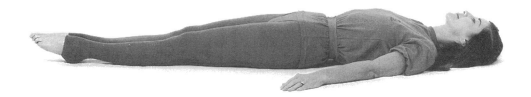

2 Bend one leg for 4 beats.

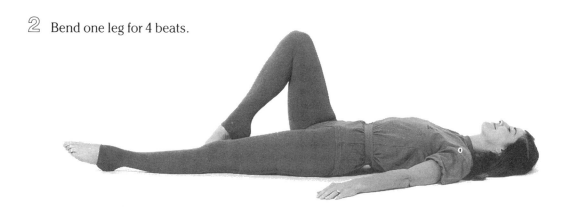

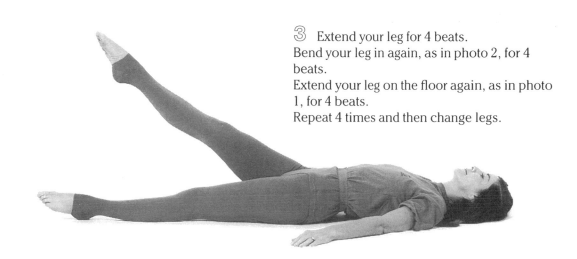

③ Extend your leg for 4 beats.
Bend your leg in again, as in photo 2, for 4 beats.
Extend your leg on the floor again, as in photo 1, for 4 beats.
Repeat 4 times and then change legs.

④ In time your leg will go higher.

When your muscles have strengthened a little, try this slightly more difficult variation of the movement.

Bend your leg and extend it, as shown in photos 2 and 3. Then lower it with the knee straight for 8 beats.
Repeat the movement 4 times and then change legs.

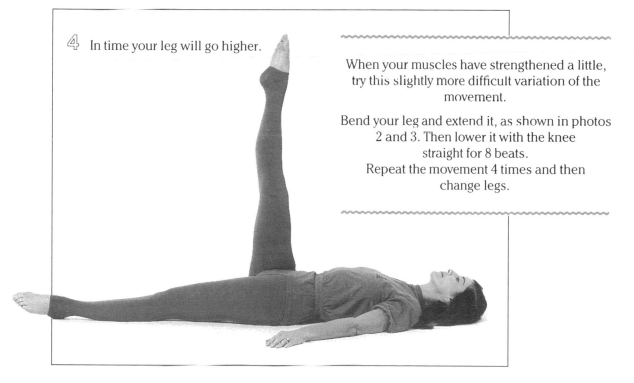

LEG WORK

BOTH LEGS

Leg Work with both legs not only strengthens, firms and slims the legs, feet and toes, but it also flattens the stomach and strengthens the back.

Just breathe normally when doing the movement.

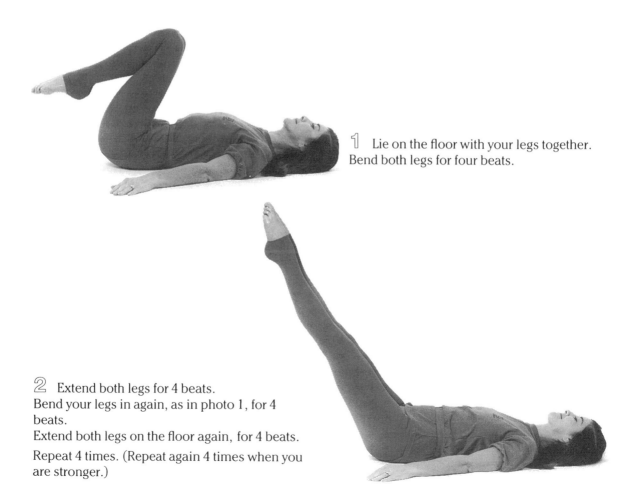

1 Lie on the floor with your legs together. Bend both legs for four beats.

2 Extend both legs for 4 beats.
Bend your legs in again, as in photo 1, for 4 beats.
Extend both legs on the floor again, for 4 beats.

Repeat 4 times. (Repeat again 4 times when you are stronger.)

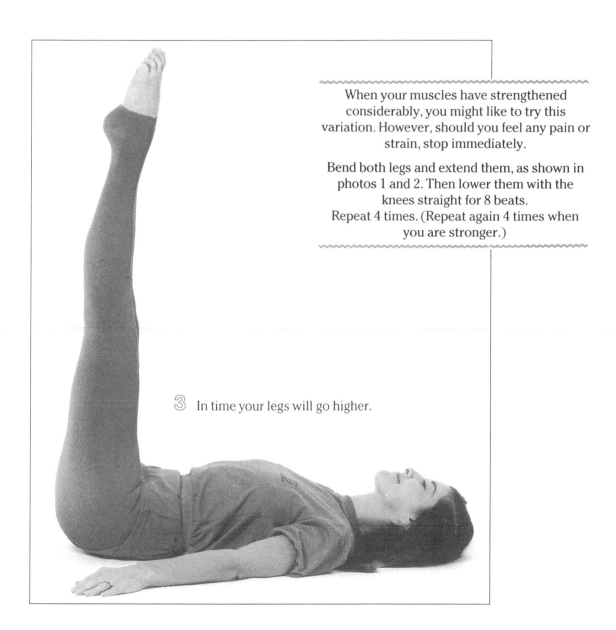

When your muscles have strengthened considerably, you might like to try this variation. However, should you feel any pain or strain, stop immediately.

Bend both legs and extend them, as shown in photos 1 and 2. Then lower them with the knees straight for 8 beats.
Repeat 4 times. (Repeat again 4 times when you are stronger.)

③ In time your legs will go higher.

SIDE RAISE

This movement slims and firms the buttocks and thighs, and strengthens the back, legs, feet and toes.

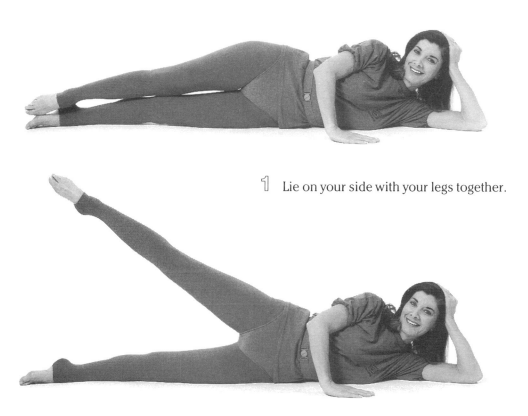

1   Lie on your side with your legs together.

2   Inhale and raise your leg for 4 beats.
Exhale and lower your leg, as in photo 1,
for 4 beats.
Repeat 8 times and then change sides.

③ In time your leg will go higher.

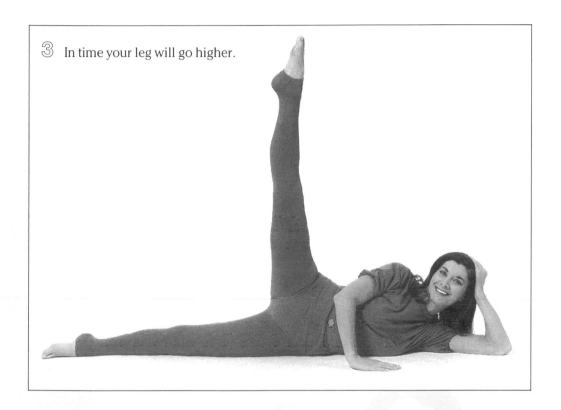

HIP TWIST

This movement slims and firms the waist, hips, buttocks and legs. It also strengthens the back and works out any stiffness and tension from the centre of the back.

Try to keep both shoulders on the floor as you do the twisting movement. Just breathe normally during the Hip Twist.

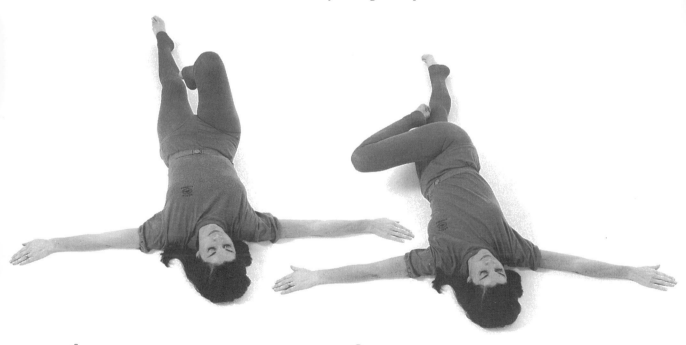

1 Lie on the floor with your legs together. Bend your right knee in for 4 beats.

2 Take the knee over to your left side for 4 beats.
Return to position 1 for 4 beats.
Slide the leg out along the floor back to your starting position for 4 beats.
Repeat on the other side and perform the movement 4 times with each leg alternately, 8 times in all.

③ When you have built up a little strength, try this variation. Bring the knee over bent as in photo 2. Extend the leg for 4 beats as shown here.

Bend it in again for 4 beats.

Return to position 1 and then slide your leg out along the floor for 4 beats.

Repeat on the other side and perform the movement 4 times with each leg alternately, 8 times in all.

LOCUST

This movement strengthens the back, and slims and firms the buttocks and hips.

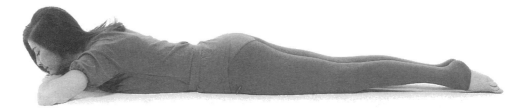

1   Lie on your stomach with your chin resting on your hands.

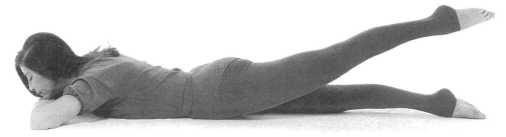

2   Inhale and raise your leg for 4 beats. Exhale and lower your leg for 4 beats. Repeat with the other leg and perform the movement 4 times with each leg alternately, 8 times in all. (Repeat again, 4 times with each leg, when you are stronger.)

③ In time you will be able to raise your leg higher.

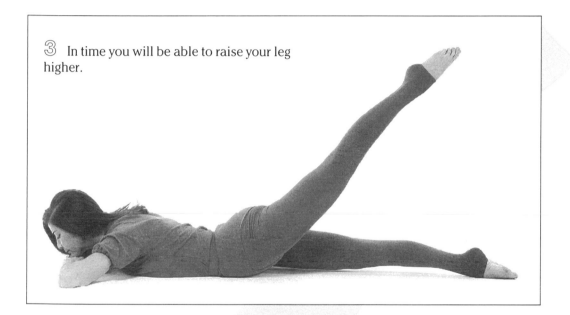

SIT UP – LIE DOWN

This simple movement conditions the entire body from head to toe. However, wait
until you have built up a little strength before you attempt it.

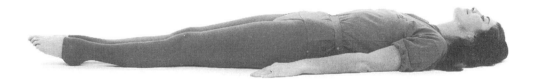

1   Lie flat on your back on the floor.

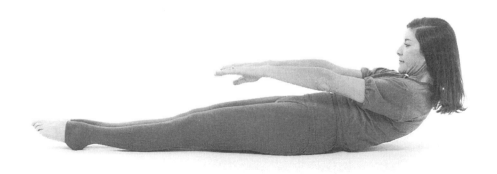

2   Inhale as you reach forwards.

③ Take 4 beats to come into this sitting position.

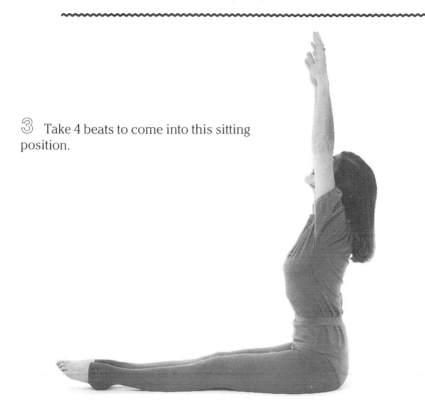

④ Roll back down again, exhaling for 4 beats. Repeat the sitting up – lying down movement 4 times. (Repeat again 4 times when you are stronger.)

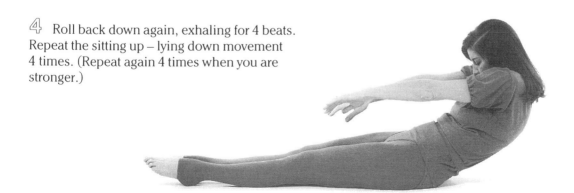

YOGACISE ROUTINES

~~~~~~~~~~~~~~~~

The following Yogacise routines have been specially formulated so that each routine will gently exercise your whole body. There are two routines for five minutes, two for ten minutes and two for fifteen minutes. Note that the timings are approximate.

Your choice of routine will depend on how much time you have available and which routine you prefer. When and if you feel like a change, simply swap to a different routine.

Feel free to replace any movement with another of your choice in any of the routines.

You may decide to alternate your routines, practising different routines on different days. Or you may wish to formulate your own routines from your favourite Yogacise movements, and that is also absolutely fine.

As many people find the standing exercises enjoyable and convenient to do, I have included a five-minute 'standing only' routine.

FIVE-MINUTE YOGACISE ROUTINES

ROUTINE A			ROUTINE B		
Standing Routine					
STANDING BREATH		21	SEATED BACK WAVE		50
STANDING REACH-UP (single arm)		22	SHOULDER TWIST		51
SQUAT		32	COIL		68
SIDE SLIDE		26	HIP PUSH		72
			FOOT WORK		61

TEN-MINUTE YOGACISE ROUTINES

ROUTINE A

STANDING REACH-UP (both arms)		24
SIDE SLIDE		26
FORWARD BEND		30
SIT DOWN		36
KNEELING BACK WAVE		37
LEG WORK (single leg)		74
FISTS		59
SHOULDER ROTATIONS		51

ROUTINE B

SEATED REACH-UP		44
HEAD TO KNEES		46
FISH		70
HIP TWIST		80
SIDE RAISE		78
LOCUST		82
'V'		42

FIFTEEN-MINUTE YOGACISE ROUTINES

ROUTINE A			ROUTINE B		
STANDING BREATH		21	STANDING REACH-UP (single arm)		22
TRIANGLE		28	STANDING REACH-UP (both arms)		24
KNEELING REACH-UP		34	SQUAT		32
UNCOIL		38	COBRA		66
'V'		42	LOCUST		82
CAT		40	LYING BREATH		62
LEG WORK (single leg)		74	ARM CIRCLING		52
HIP TWIST		80	ELBOW BENDS		53
HIP PUSH		72	FINGER SPREAD		58
STRETCH		64	HEAD ROLL		54
SHOULDER ROTATIONS		51	EYE ROTATIONS		56

YOGACISE AND PREGNANCY

~~~~~~~~~~~~~~~~~~~~

The practice of Yogacise is a wonderful way of keeping fit both during pregnancy and after your baby is born.

 The following movements are particularly recommended for the duration of your pregnancy, but any movements not included in this list are best avoided. Once your baby is born, you can safely practise all of the Yogacise movements.

Yogacise Standing Breath	21
Yogacise Standing Reach-Up (single arm)	22
Yogacise Standing Reach-Up (both arms)	24
Yogacise Side Slide	26
Yogacise Triangle	28
Yogacise Squat	32
Yogacise Kneeling Reach-Up	34
Yogacise Sit down	36
Yogacise Kneeling Back Wave	37
Yogacise Cat	40
Yogacise Seated Reach-Up	44
Yogacise Shoulder Twist	48
Yogacise Shoulder Rotations	51
Yogacise Arm Circling	52
Yogacise Elbow Bends	53
Yogacise Head Roll	54
Yogacise Eye Rotations	56
Yogacise Finger Spread	58
Yogacise Fists	59
Yogacise Finger Pulls	60
Yogacise Foot Work	61
Yogacise Lying Breath	62
Yogacise Stretch	64
Yogacise Fish	70
Yogacise Leg Work (single leg)	74

GLOSSARY

〜〜〜〜〜〜〜〜

Practice of the Yogacise movements brings many physical, mental and emotional benefits. Listed below are all the Yogacise movements with details of the particular benefits that they bring.

Yogacise Standing Breath   Page 21
Strengthens the back, shoulders and arms.
Improves breathing.
Very relaxing.

Yogacise Standing Reach-Up (single arm)   Page 22
Stretches and firms the sides of the body.
Strengthens the back, shoulders, arms and hands.

Yogacise Standing Reach-Up (both arms)   Page 24
Stretches the back and the sides.
Flattens and firms the stomach.
Strengthens the back, shoulders, arms and hands.

Yogacise Side Slide   Page 26
Stretches the sides of the body.
Slims the waist.
Strengthens the back.
Improves balance.

Yogacise Triangle   Page 28
Stretches, slims and firms the sides of the body and the upper arms.
Strengthens the back, shoulders and legs.
Improves balance and co-ordination.

Yogacise Forward Bend   Page 30
Stretches and strengthens the back and neck.
Relaxes the neck, shoulders, arms and hands.
Improves the complexion.
Revitalising.
Very relaxing.

Glossary

Yogacise Squat　Page 32
Strengthens the legs and back.
Slims, firms and tones the thighs.
The variations shown also strengthen the shoulders and the arms.

Yogacise Kneeling Reach-Up　Page 34
Slims and firms the thighs, waist and stomach.
Strengthens the back, shoulders, arms and hands.
Stretches the back and the sides of the body.

Yogacise Sit Down　Page 36
Firms and slims the buttocks, tummy and thighs.
Strengthens the back, shoulders and arms.

Yogacise Kneeling Back Wave　Page 37
Increases strength and suppleness in the back and neck.
Very relaxing.

Yogacise Uncoil　Page 38
Increases strength and flexibility in the back.
Flattens the stomach.

Yogacise Cat　Page 40
Increases strength and flexibility throughout the back and neck.
Firm and slims the buttocks, hips, waist and stomach.
Strengthens the shoulders, arms and wrists.
Relieves tension and stiffness in the neck and shoulder area.

Yogacise 'V'　Page 42
Stretches the back and the legs.
Strengthens the toes, ankles, shoulders, arms and wrists.
Slims and firms the thighs.
Improves the complexion.
Refreshes and revitalises.

Yogacise Seated Reach-Up　Page 44
Strengthens the back, shoulders, arms and hands.
Stretches and firms the sides of the body.
Firms and slims the legs.

Glossary

Yogacise Head to Knees   Page 46
Stretches the neck and back.
Relieves tension and stiffness from those areas.
Position 4 also stretches the backs of the legs.

Yogacise Shoulder Twist   Page 48
Slims and firms the waist.
Strengthens the back, shoulders, neck and arms.

Yogacise Seated Back Wave   Page 50
Increases strength and suppleness in the back and neck.
Strengthens the shoulders, arms and wrists.

Yogacise Shoulder Rotations   Page 51
Relieves stiffness and tension from the shoulders, neck and top of the back.
Relaxing and good for releasing stress.

Yogacise Arm Circling   Page 52
Strengthens the arms, shoulders and back.

Yogacise Elbow Bends   Page 53
Works the elbow joints to keep them strong and healthy.
Strengthens the shoulders and arms.

Yogacise Head Roll   Page 54
Relieves stiffness and tension from the neck and top of the back.
Gently stretches the neck.
Very relaxing.

Yogacise Eye Rotations   Page 56
Works the eye muscles to keep them healthy.

Yogacise Finger Spread   Page 58
Strengthens the fingers, hands and arms.
Releases tension and stress generally.

Yogacise Fists   Page 59
Strengthens the hands and arms.
Releases tension and stress generally.

Glossary

Yogacise Finger Pulls Page 60
Works on the finger joints to keep them healthy.
Strengthens the top of the back, shoulders, arms and wrists.
Develops the chest muscles.

Yogacise Foot Work Page 61
Strengthens the feet and toes.
Slims the ankies.
Strengthens and firms the legs.

Yogacise Lying Breath Page 62
Improves breathing generally.
Gives the body a gentle overall stretch.

Yogacise Stretch Page 64
Gives the body a good head-to-toe stretch.
Firms and strengthens the entire body.
Improves breathing generally.
Removes tension and stress, and is very relaxing.

Yogacise Cobra Page 66
Strengthens the back and the neck, increasing suppleness.
Strengthens the shoulders, arms and wrists.
Relieves stiffness and tension in the neck and top of the back.

Yogacise Coil Page 68
Stretches and strengthens the back and the neck, promoting flexibility.
Strengthens the shoulders, arms, wrists and fingers.
Relieves stiffness and tension from the neck area.

Yogacise Fish Page 70
Increases strength and suppleness in the back.
Strengthens the neck, shoulders and arms.
Improves the complexion.
Very relaxing.

Yogacise Hip Push Page 72
Strengthens the centre of the back.
Firms and slims the thighs and buttocks.

Glossary

Yogacise Leg Work (single leg)   Page 74
Strengthens the legs, feet and toes.
Slims and firms the thighs and calves.

Yogacise Leg Work (both legs)   Page 76
Strengthens the legs, feet, toes and back.
Firms and slims the thighs and calves.
Flattens and firms the stomach.

Yogacise Side Raise   Page 78
Slims and firms the buttocks and thighs.
Strengthens the back, legs, feet and toes

Yogacise Hip Twist   Page 80
Slims and firms the waist, hips, buttocks and legs.
Strengthens the back.
Relieves stiffness and tension from the centre of the back.

Yogacise Locust   Page 82
Strengthens the back.
Slims and firms the buttocks, legs and hips.

Yogacise Sit Up – Lie Down   Page 84
Slims and firms the entire body from head to toe.